Plant Based Eating

The Beginner's Guide to Energize Your Body and Kickstart Your Healthy Lifestyle Eating Green

Gwenda Flores

Table of contents

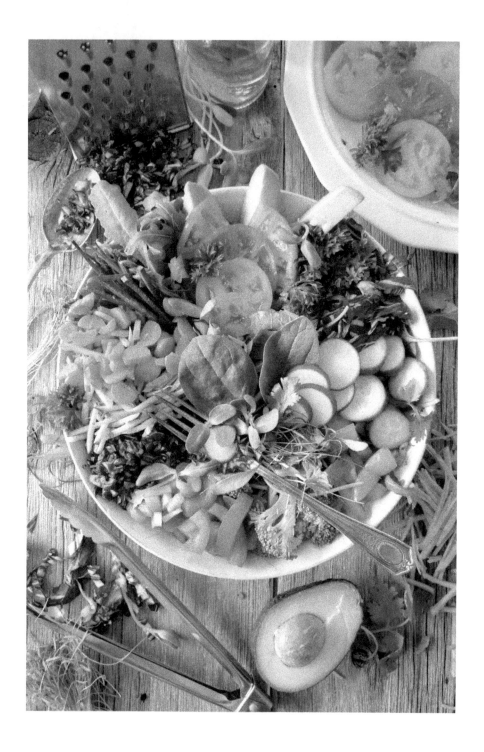

INTRODUCTION

As our society evolves, we are constantly facing the need to change our behaviours and habits to increase our health and quality of life. We are now facing climate change, food insecurity and over 40% of population is suffering from chronic disease. One of recent ideas want to improve our world and health is the plant-based nutrition. Even though food regiments are not something our doctor prescribes (yet), research is showing that food has a lot to contribute to our health. It is also a less costly option to our society than prescribing medication. Whether you want to save the animals, become healthier or simply feel good and better, plant-based nutrition is a great option for those of us who want to be a better and healthier person. Choosing a plant-based nutrition is not a complex commitment.

With the help of this guide, you will be ready to step into the world of plant-based eating in no time and set yourself up for success. You will learn about plant-based nutrition, much research about it and how to easily and successfully transition into a plant-based nutrition.

You will find some recipes to kick-start your journey and find answers to questions might be limiting you in your transition to a plant-based diet. Let's define what plant-based eating is all about.

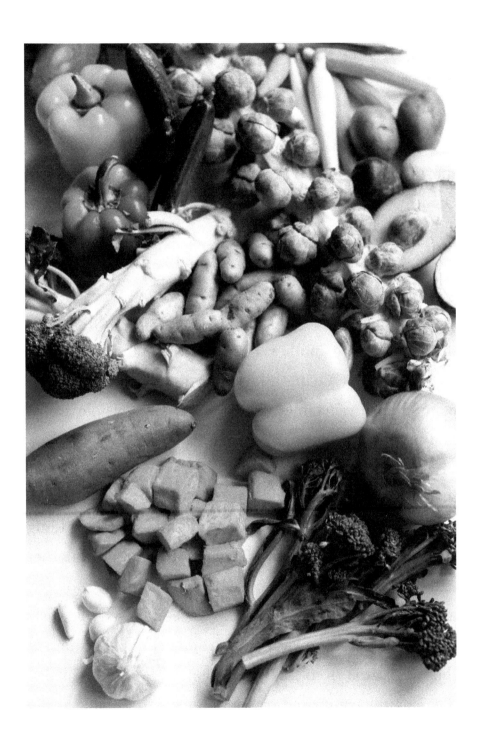

CHAPTER 1: WHAT IS PLANT-BASED EATING?

We are hearing the word plant-based nutrition more and more in our society. With the launch of documentaries like Game Changers, books like Forks over knives and the emergence of athletes changing their nutrition to be plant-based, one must wonder what this is all about.

Our understanding of plant-based eating may differ from one individual to another. In the world of nutrition, plant-based eating is having a large portion of one's nutrition coming from vegetables, fruits, herbs, nuts, whole grains and include legumes or other plants.

A spectrum of plant-based nutrition options is available to you. Some are very strict (vegan diet), others are adding animal products like dairy (vegetarian) and, at the other end of the spectrum, are those that still eat meat, poultry, and fish on an occasional basis. We once believed that early humans consumed a large proportion of animal protein in their diet. It is from that belief that, in the 2000s, Paleo diet (mainly comprised of animal protein) became really popular in the world of nutrition and diet.

Although, we now know that nutrition of bipedal primates and Homo sapiens was primarily composed of nuts, fruits, leaves, roots, seeds, and water. In that case, the "original" Paleo Diet was plant-based eating. It is also linked to the fact that some of the strongest animals on Earth are not carnivores. The strongest mammal is the gorilla (most are herbivores animals). It can lift around 4409 lbs., that is ten times its body weight. It would be like a 200 lb. individual lifting 2000 lb. If other mammals can live a healthy and strong life on a plant-based nutrition, we probably can too.

Why choose a plant-based nutrition?

Many reasons exist for choosing a plant-based nutrition, we will discuss in more details some of those reasons but here is our top 5:

1) Improve your physical health:
Most people consume double recommended daily intake of protein which can also cause issues with digestion.
Reducing your intake of animal food, you will most likely reach the recommended daily intake of protein without surpassing it.

In addition, an increased consumption of grains, beans, fruits and vegetables can bring more fiber into your daily nutrition. Most Americans do not consume enough fiber and that can lead to inflammation of the digestive tract, constipation and hemorrhoids.

2) Succeed in weight loss and weight management:

In general, individuals who are on a plant-based nutrition, tend to consume fewer calories than who consume animal protein. That is because most of their calories are coming from healthier options and fewer calories per weight. Plant-based eaters tend to eat less process food and avoid meat focused restaurants like fast-food chain that provide unhealthy meal options.

3) Prevent or manage a chronic disease:

As you will see in next section, research demonstrates that individuals on a plant-based nutrition can prevent chronic disease, reduce obesity, and mostly encourage a healthy lifestyle and increase their quality of life.

4) Stop spending on supplements:

Did you know that our nation's population spends more than $30 billion a year on supplements? What if you did not need to waste that money? With plant-based nutrition, you are more likely to receive all nutrients you need from natural sources like legumes, vegetables, and fruits. Not only does this save you money, but it also saves you from trying to remember to purchase, consume supplements.

5) Save our planet:

Agriculture uses approximately 70% of fresh water on our planet (globally on average). That said, the production of meat requires around 1000% more water (1 kg requires from 5000 to 20,000 liters of water) than some grains like wheat (1 kg of wheat requires between 500 and 4000 liters of water). In addition, a lot of grain is cultivated to feed the animals we eat and if we started eating grain and reduce our consumption of meat, less water and fewer resources would be used to produce animal food.

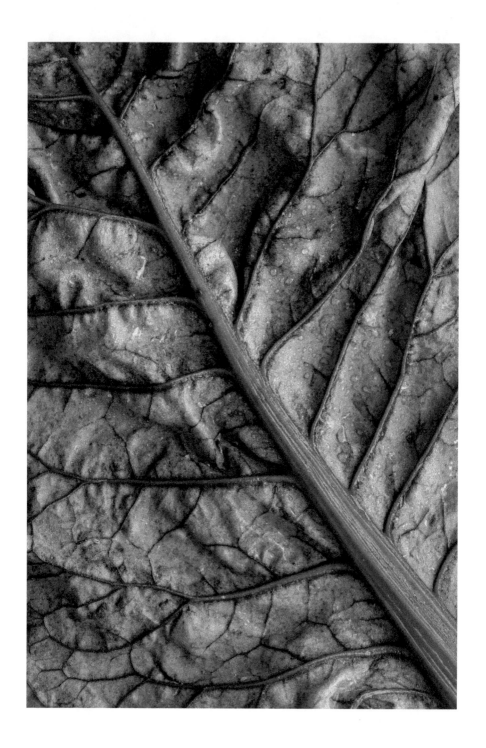

CHAPTER 2: THE SCIENCE BEHIND PLANT-BASED EATING

Plant-based diet is simply a dietary scheme predominantly prefers foods of plant origin. The purposes are different: to lose weight in primis, and to heal. Many people even link this diet to cancer prevention but - as we are talking about an extremely serious subject - we urge you not to take literally what is written, nor to try do it yourself remedies.

Go to a specialist or a nutritionist, always, but even more so if you are involved in serious pathologies and want to understand if and how food can be involved in a path of wellness. Some sources use positive research conducted by Harvard medical School. How does plant-based diet work? Simply, it plays on the fact that vegetables, fruits and herbs should always be the main food during main meals.

The prevalence of foods of plant origin therefore brings in the background the presence of meat and foods of animal origin: milk, eggs, cheese, fish, white meat, but especially red meat are extremely reduced in a monthly overview.

The *red meat=cancer* argument has been going around for years and many figures (including doctors) have confirmed a correlation. However, it is never a smart and productive move to generalize and only a serious nutritionist should set the consumption on our physical needs.

As already mentioned, several medical-scientific realities have demonstrated that a high and regular consumption of vegetable foods has a decisive role in reducing the risk of many problems, even serious ones: metabolic syndrome, cardiovascular diseases, concrete help in cases of a high blood pressure, prevention of cancer and diabetes.

Reducing or avoiding meat and fish at times does not mean becoming vegetarian or vegan. Vegetarian and vegan diets have quite different origins and are also above all based on ethical principles of consumption. The message brought by the herbal data is not to avoid meat like the plague, but that it could be a healthy solution to simply get used to eat much less of it: it brings the example of the Mediterranean diet, a scheme which prefers legumes and vegetables to fish and meat.

The plant diet is also based on balancing them in the right way, vegetables and fruits can provide all the necessary nutrients: proteins, carbohydrates, fats. Here you can find the rules to follow:

- Fill at least half your plate with vegetables, both at lunch and dinner.
- Choose only good fats for seasoning: avocado, cold-pressed extra virgin olive oil, oily seeds.
- Vary and involve all "colors" of vegetables and fruits (there is even a diet of colors).
- Replace sweets with fruit.
- Drastically reduce consumption of meat, both red or white.

Research shows that we need more fruits and vegetables in our plates to prevent chronic disease and help with our weight management. In next chapter, you will learn about what we need more in our nutrition intake (fruits, fiber and vegetables) and what we need less (sodium, sugar, protein) to live a healthier life.

Fruits and Vegetables

Plant-based eating means that you have a large proportion of your meal that comes from plant-based food. That said, fruits and vegetables are often the number one thing that comes to mind when we think of a plant-based nutrition. According to some studies, only 15% of our population can meet the minimum requirement of daily recommendation for fruits and even less (10%) for vegetables. Experts in nutrition - across the world - agree that an insufficient consumption of fruits and vegetables contribute to the obesity epidemic and chronic disease related to poor nutrition, especially in our country.

A report published by World Health Organization (WHO) recommended that a daily intake of 400 g of fruits and vegetable would contribute to preventing chronic diseases which include diabetes, heart disease, cancer, and obesity. To put this in perspective, one tomato is approximately 75 g while a medium size potato is about 150 grams. For fruits, a medium apple is about 150 g and a small kiwi is around 75 g.

Fiber

As mentioned earlier, fiber is lacking in the nutrition of Americans. It is recommended to consume from 25 g (women) to 38 g (men) of fiber daily. Unfortunately, we consume an average of 15 g daily. That is not enough for most of us and can have a negative impact on the bowels and cause constipation or hemorrhoids.

According to research, an increase intake in fiber can help prevent and reduce heart diseases, diabetes, and colon cancer. You can find two types of fiber, water-soluble and water insoluble. Water-soluble fiber can be found in fruits, vegetables, legumes, oat, and bran. Since water-soluble fiber absorbs water during digestion, it can help decrease or prevent constipation.

Fiber is also known to decrease blood cholesterol levels. As for water-insoluble fibers, they can be found in vegetables, fruits, whole grains and cereals, including brown rice. The insoluble fiber wears that name because they remain. Unchanged during the digestion and help with digestion, encouraging a regular movement in the intestine.

Here is the approximate amount of fiber found in various plant-based foods:

- ½ cup of black beans, 7 g
- ½ cup of cooked broccoli, 5 g
- 1 apple, 4 g
- ½ cup Bran cereal (no sugar), 14 g
- 1 cup cooked brown rice, 3.5 g
- 1 cup of oatmeal, 4 g

Sodium

Sodium might be considered a plant-based food but there is a strong warning to decrease our consumption so that we do not exceed the requirements of 2300 mg of sodium consumption daily. Saltshaker in your kitchen is rarely the culprit. Sodium usually comes from highly processed foods (frozen aisle in grocery store) and restaurant meals.

For example, a fast-food burger can have twice the sodium a homemade one has. According to research, individuals who regularly consume a meal at fast-food restaurants were approximately 296 mg above recommended daily intake.

Other studies indicate that individuals who had a plant-based nutrition with reduce sodium consumption (2300-1500 mg per day) showed a reduction in the blood pressure and increased weight loss. That said, is important to understand that plant-based food does not always mean healthy food. Sugar is other plant-based food to beware of.

Sugar

Did you know we are among the largest sugar producers in the world? And we are also high consumers of sugar (3rd country in the world after India and China). The average American will consume 152 pounds (six 25 lb. bags of sugar cane) of sugar a year. Some people will try to convince you that some sugars are better than others. It is true that different types of sugars will have a different impact on your metabolism. But sugar remains something that you should not consume in a large quantity no matter if it is coming from fruit juices, honey, or a muffin.

It is recommended to stick to less than 50 g of sugar a day. A packet of sugar is about 4 g, one glass of cow milk is about 14 g of sugar, a popular brand of store-bought muffin is approximately 32 g of sugar added.

We challenge you to start looking at the labels of the food you eat daily and identify the amount of sugar intake you get from those foods. You will be quickly surprised to see that sugar is added to so many products we purchase. Even canned vegetables can have added sugar. By reducing your sugar intake, you increase your chance of losing weights and staying healthy while preventing chronic disease. Reading labels can be difficult, look for the word sugar on the nutrition label, you will see how many grams of sugar there is in the product. Many companies hide ingredient by using multiple names to describe the sugar added, they use at least 60 names for sugar on labels.

Companies do it that way because they can "divide and conquer" if they only used name sugar, it would often be one of first ingredients on the list (which is in order of quantity) and that would tell us that it is not a healthy option. To confuse you (even more) into submission, they categorize the type of sugar by its scientific name so that they can have ten small amounts of sugar instead of one large amount of sugar. Here is an example, the order of ingredients on a popular can of pumpkin pie filling reads like this: pumpkin, water, sugar, salt, spices, dextrose and natural flavours.

Dextrose is a type of sugar, and some companies chose to use that term instead of sugar because it would have placed sugar before pumpkin in the ingredient list. Same with a popular bottle of our ketchup that has the following ingredient label: tomato concentrate from ripe red tomatoes, corn syrup, distilled vinegar, high-fructose corn syrup, onion powder, salt, spice, natural flavouring. This one uses the term high-fructose corn syrup and corn syrup to describe sugar. One packet of ketchup weighs 9 g and 2 g is sugar.

I know, choosing healthy seems like a lot of work, but once you know which products are good for you, it makes your grocery shopping quicker. Some labels now say low sodium or no sugar added, this can help you pick the right item faster.

Protein

It is a myth that animal protein is a better protein than plant protein. Since 2007, the World Health Organization has indicated that the difference between animal or plant-based protein is not significant.

Here some examples of approximate amount of the protein found in plant-based protein versus animal protein:

Plant-based Protein

1 cup of dry roasted soy, 37 g

1 cup of tofu, 20 g

1 cup of boiled chickpeas, 15 g

1 cup of quinoa, 8 g

1 avocado, 4 g

Animal Protein

1 Ribeye steak (291 g), 69 g

1 fillet of cooked salmon, 35 g

1 cup of cottage cheese, 23 g

1 cup of whole milk, 8 g

1 egg, 6 g

For most Americans, the average daily intake of protein is recommended at 46 g (women) and 56 g (men). One cup of shredded cheese is about 26 g of protein and a 1 cup of diced chicken is 38 g of protein.

That means that if you eat cottage cheese for breakfast with a glass of milk, an egg sandwich for lunch, and ribeye steak for dinner, you are probably looking at double amount of protein recommend for daily intake. You can understand why the average American eat around 100 g of protein per day. Our society seems to be eating too much protein, which can cause issues with the bowels or digestion. It is true that some individuals need more protein than others but in general, our protein rich nutrition is overindulgence.

It was once believed that you needed to add animal protein in your meals to increase muscle mass. Some studies and athletes have demonstrated that it is possible to increase muscles and be strong and fit with a plant-based nutrition. An example? One of the best runners of ever and American ultramarathoner, Scott Jurek, is known to be a plant-based eater!

While thousands of researches, demonstrate health benefit of consuming vegetables, fruits to prevent illness, many still refuse to change their nutrition to increase quality of life. Too many people believe that exercising, medication and supplements are sufficient to maintain health.

Meanwhile, experts in the field of health and wellness say that weight management is 75–80% nutrition and 20–25% exercise. So why do we still struggle to implement change? What stops you from applying the changes to your life? Well, there is a saying that some people only change when status quo is more uncomfortable than changing. Are you that kind of person? Are you really waiting for your health to be gone to make your illness your number one priority? I do not think so, because you would not be reading this if you were not contemplating a change. Since you are not a quitter, let's move on to next chapter. We will be making sure that you have all the tools and knowledge to reach your plant-based eating goal with success!

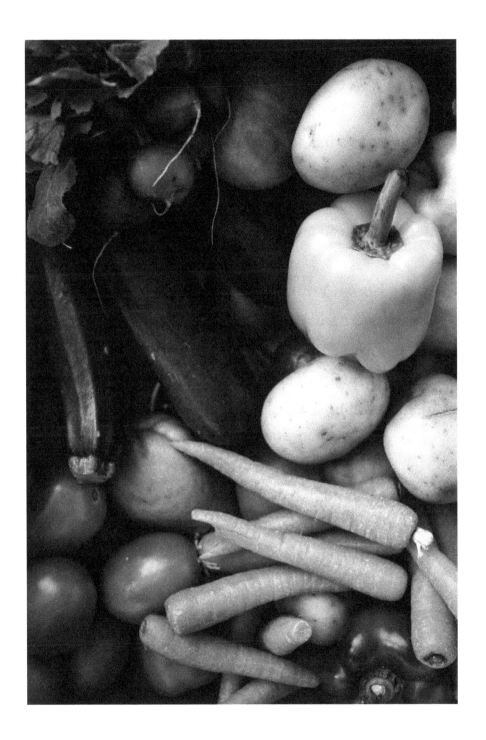

CHAPTER 3: KICKSTART YOUR PLANT-BASED LIFESTYLE

To be successful in adopting a good plant-based lifestyle, it is recommended to take small steps so that you can adopt and maintain your new habits. Slow and steady is a great strategy to form new habits.

Step 1: Choose Your Type of Plant-Based Nutrition
As mentioned earlier, a spectrum of plant-based eating is available to you. Start by identifying what you would like to change in your nutrition. Considering your nutrition will be mainly coming from plants, your options are:

1) Strict plant-based nutrition (vegan): With a strict plant-based nutrition, you are not going to consume any meat, fish or animal products like dairy foods, honey, or eggs.

2) Vegetarian plant-based nutrition: In a plant-based nutrition, you will be able to consume eggs, milk, cheese and other products of animals but no meat or fish.

3) Pescatarian plant-based nutrition: The pescatarian plant-based nutrition is like the vegetarian one but include fish. That would mean that your nutrition includes plant-base food, eggs, milk, cheese, fish and other products of animals but no meat.

4) Flexitarian plant-based nutrition: It is great for who would like to slowly move into plant-based eating without fully committing to never eat meat again. In this plant-based nutrition option, your meals will have a large proportion of plant-base food. In addition to small portions of eggs, or dairy foods and, on occasion, include meat, fish, seafood, and poultry. Some people in that category have adopted the meatless Mondays to reduce their consumption of animal protein.

Is it hard for you to decide? If is like this, let me ask you this question. On a scale of 1 (not ready) to 10 (let's do this), how ready are you to make a change in your nutrition? If you said 1-5, try option 4. But if you said 6-10, try option 2 and see if you can stick to it. Maybe give yourself a month to ease into your new change.

For example, stop purchasing meat products when you go to grocery, finish eating all the animal food in the fridge and freezer. We do not want to cause food waste, especially if you are choosing plant-based eating for environmental benefits.

Step 2: Adapt Your Grocery

To ease yourself into plant-based eating, try to slowly increase the amount of plant-based food on your grocery list, stop purchasing animal protein and dairy products. Stock up on cans of legumes such as chickpeas, black beans since they are fast and easy ingredients to add to many recipes (just make sure they are not full of sugar or salt).

When purchasing vegetables in cans instead of selecting fresh ones, make sure to read the label and avoid added sugar or salt. You can pick a no- or low-sodium option. In addition, you can also select frozen vegetables like peas or corn, the same warning applies. Make sure to read the label, some frozen food has added sugar, salt and butter. You can start by looking at the labels on the products that you have in your pantry and freezer.

This might require a bit more shopping time at first but eventually, you will know which brand is the healthiest for you. Here are some examples of items that could be on your plant-based grocery list:

Fruits	Vegetables	
Apples	Asparagus	Sweet
Apricot	Avocado	Peppers
Bananas	Beets	Jalapenos
Blackberries	Bok Choy	Chilis
Blueberries	Broccoli	Potatoes
Cantaloupe	Brussels sprouts	Spinach
Cherries	Carrots	Squash
Grapefruit	Cauliflower	Zucchini
Grapes	Celery	Sweet
Honeydew	Corn	potatoes
Kiwis	Cucumbers	
Lemons/Limes	Eggplant	
Nectarines	Garlic	
Oranges	Green beans	
Peaches	Lettuce/Greens	
Pears	Mushrooms	
Plums	Okra	
Raspberries	Onions	
Strawberries	Squash	
Kiwis	Spinach	
Watermelon	Tomatoes	

Grains	Legumes and nuts	Herbs and spices	Other
Basmati Rice	Chickpeas	Basil	Vegan sour
Jasmine Rice	Pinto	Black	cream
Brown Rice	Beans	pepper	Vegan
White Rice	Lentils	Bay leaf	mayonnaise
Wild Rice	Split Peas	Cilantro	Vegan bread
Arborio Rice	Mung	Cinnamon	& wraps
(Orzo)	beans	Cumin	Whole grain
Farro	Red	Curry	mustard
Quinoa	kidney	Garlic	Bran cereals
Tabbouleh	beans	Ginger	Honey
Couscous	Soy	Mint	Maple syrup
Barley	beans	Oregano	Peanut
Rolled Oat	Black	Paprika	butter
Steel Cut Oat	beans	Parsley	Almond milk
	White	Red	Coconut milk
	beans	pepper	Coconut oil
	Pecans	Salt	Olive oil
	Cashews	Turmeric	Hummus
	Peanuts	Vanilla	Tahini
	Walnuts	extract	
	Alfalfa		
	Sprouts		
	Carob		

Step 3: Plan your meals

One of the most difficult parts about adapting to plant-based eating is to adopt new habits in the kitchen. Instead of having burgers or roasted chicken for dinner, you must find new ways to cook and bring more plant-based food at your table. If you are going to try the vegan approach, breakfast might be the most difficult to adapt, especially if you are used to eat eggs in the morning.

It is strongly recommended to try new recipes as opposed to try to adapt your old recipes to a plant-based nutrition. For example, a plant-based Mac and Cheese is hard to make. In the regular dish, cheese is the main ingredient and plant-based cheese is far from having the same taste and texture.

Here are a few ideas of meals you can plan for each meal. If you are going for the strict plant-based nutrition, make sure to select items that are vegan-friendly for the bread, wraps, mayonnaise, and other condiments.

Breakfast

Breakfast can be difficult when you are used to a bacon and egg type of breakfast. Try to keep fruits, bran cereal and oat, and vegan bread in the house, that way, you will have quick options when you do not want to think too much about what to make. Here are some breakfast ideas:

- Bran cereals with bananas and plant-base milk (this will be a winner for your fiber intake).
- Oatmeal in a jar (see recipe in the next chapter)
- Vegan bread with natural peanut butter, no sugar added jam
- Fruit salad
- Hummus and pita bread

Lunch

If your usual lunch is deli meat sandwiches, you will be going through a bit of a transition for meal planning. In general, many plant-based options can be quick and made in advance (i.e., salad in a jar). In the next chapter, you will find recipes of salads, wraps and soups that you can make for your lunch.

Dinner

In general, dinner is the time when individuals spent more time with friends or families. A plant-based dinner can be a combination of vegetables, grains and legumes. Here are a few examples:

- Veggie Burger with sweet potato fries
- Vegetable, black beans and rice stir fry
- Rice and beans with plantains (see next chapter)
- Grain bowls
- Risotto with roasted vegetables

Step 4: Let's do this!

The best way to start the plant-based eating is to start with small steps now. Choose a day this week when you want to have a plant-based nutrition. That day will be beginning of your journey in plant-based eating. Once you have chosen a date, pick your recipes! This next chapter will give you a few ideas of recipes you can start with.

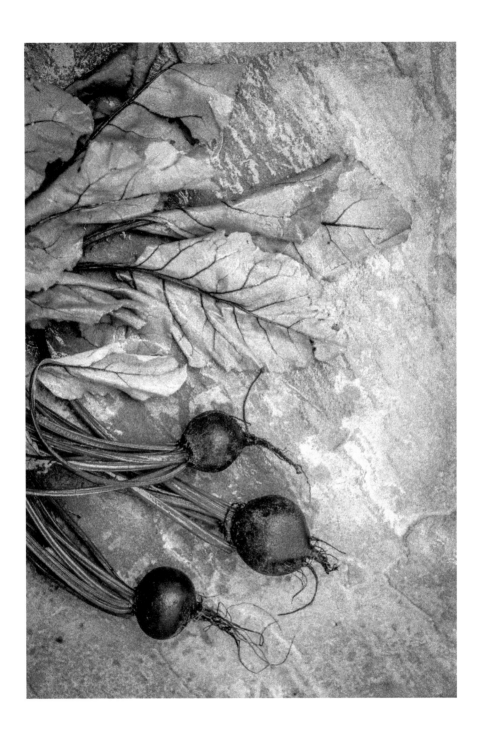

CHAPTER 4: BREAKFAST RECIPES

Kick-start your plant-based eating journey, the following recipes you can add to your meal plan.

Overnight Oatmeal

This is a great recipe that can be prepared in advance.

If you work Monday-Friday, you can prepare five jars on Sunday, keep them in the fridge and eat one before going to work. It is a great "Grab and Go" breakfast recipe, that will please everyone, even the kids!

Ingredients (for one serving)
- Mason Jar
- 2/3 cup Old-fashioned oats rolled oat or steel-cut oat
- 1 cup plant-based milk
- 1/4 teaspoon vanilla extract
- 1/4 cup frozen blueberries or frozen strawberries

- Instructions:
- Mix the vanilla and the milk in a separate bowl.
- Place the oat in the mason jar.
- Add the milk and vanilla mixed.

- Add the frozen fruits.
- Place in the jar in fridge and leave overnight (can be stored in the fridge for up to five days).

Additional tips:
- You can replace the frozen fruits with fresh fruits; if you are using bananas, it is recommended to add to the jar just before eating.
- Other toppings: coconut, peanut butter, and cinnamon.
- Want something sweeter? Adding dry dates is a great way to add some sweetness to this recipe. For healthier options, make sure the date does not include added sugar. Maple syrup or honey is another way to add fewer processed sweeteners.

Potato Breakfast Bowl

The potato breakfast bowl is a very hearty breakfast for days when you want something a little bit more filling.

Ingredients (for two serving):
- Bowl
- 3 large red potato

- 1 tablespoon of olive oil
- 1 teaspoon of garlic powder
- 1 teaspoon of chili powder
- 1 teaspoon of sea salt
- ½ of a red onion
- ½ of a green pepper
- 1 avocado, sliced
- 6 cherry tomatoes, halved

Dressing:
- ½ cup of vegan mayonnaise
- Juice from ½ a lemon
- 1 teaspoon of whole grain mustard

Instructions:
- Preheat the oven to 425 degrees.
- Clean potatoes (do not peel them) and dice them into 1" cubes.
- In a bowl, toss potatoes, olive oil and spices.
- Place on a baking sheet and bake for 30–35 minutes until browned and tender.
- In the meantime, dice the onions and peppers.

- Add the onions and peppers when 10 minutes is left to the potatoes.
- While the ingredients are roasting, you can make the dressing. In a bowl, mix the Mayo, the lemon juice and the mustard until the sauce is creamy.
- When vegetables are roasted, divide into 2 portions. Place them in a serving bowl and add sliced avocado and cherry tomatoes on top of the vegetables and serve with the dressing on top.

Additional tips:
- For the dressing, you can control the amount of lemon juice you add to make it thicker or more liquid.
- Like it spicy? Add ingredients like chilis, sriracha sauce or jalapenos to the recipe.

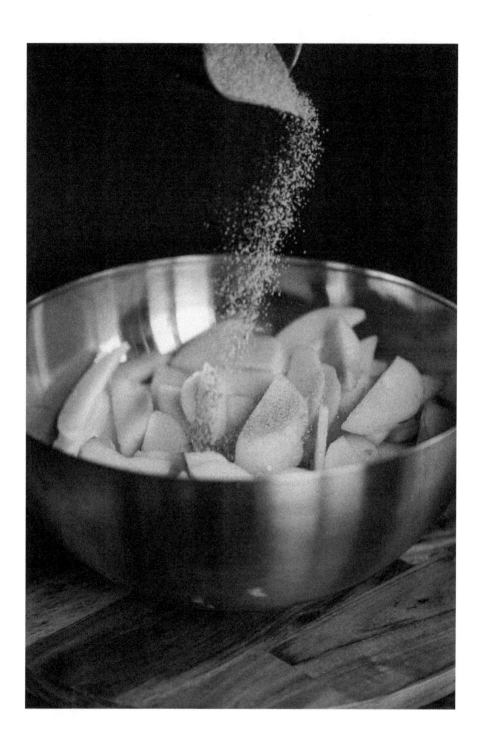

The simpleton

This recipe is for days that you feel like eating a quick and easy breakfast.

Ingredients (1 serving):
- 1 slice of vegan bread
- Peanut butter
- 1 banana, sliced
- Maple Syrup or Honey

Instructions:
- Toast the slice of bread, spread with peanut butter, add the banana slices on top and drizzle with maple syrup or honey. Eat.

Additional tip:
- Do not you like bananas? No problem! Switch the bananas for strawberries or raspberries.

Whole Grain Pancakes With Cashew Butter

Ingredients (2 servings):
- 1 cup Kodiak Cakes Buttermilk Flapjack and Waffle Mix
- 1 cup Pacific Foods Unsweetened Hemp Original beverage
- 2 Tbsp cashew butter
- 1/2 cup blueberries
- 1/2 cup strawberries
- 2 Tbsp honey

Instructions:
- Whisk pancake mix and the hemp beverage in a medium bowl until lump-free.
- Heat a seasoned cast-iron skillet over medium-high heat and pour in 1/2 cup pancake mix.
- When the pancake starts to bubble, about 3 minutes, flip over and cook for another minute.
- Place a dollop of nut butter on top of each pancake and make a stack.
- Top the stack with berries, and drizzle with honey.

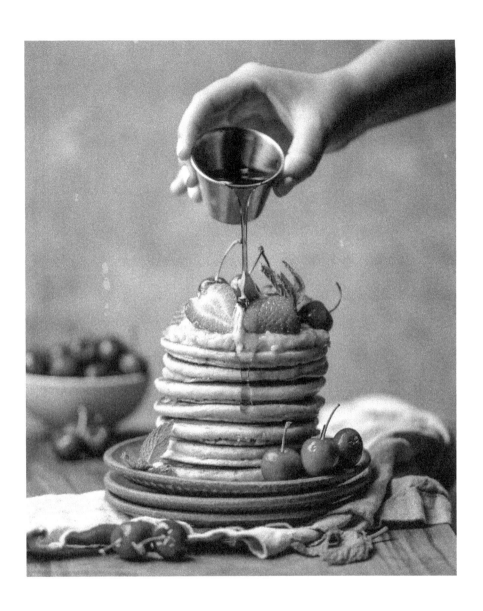

Plant-Based Lentil and Kale Tots Casserole

Ingredients (8 servings):
- 1 tsp extra virgin olive oil
- 1/4 cup minced white onion
- 1/4 tsp garlic powder
- 1/8 tsp ground thyme
- 1/8 tsp ground sage
- 1/8 tsp ground fennel
- 1/2 tsp kosher salt
- 1/8 tsp freshly ground black pepper
- 1/4 tsp ground cayenne
- One 14-oz can lentils, drained and rinsed
- 1/2 tsp maple syrup
- 1 cup shredded extra sharp cheddar cheese
- 3/4 cup whole milk
- 3 large eggs
- 2 packets Dr Praegers frozen kale puffs
- Chives, for garnish
- Hot sauce, for servin

Instructions:
- Preheat oven to 350°F.
- In a 10-inch cast iron skillet, heat the oil and cook onion, garlic powder, thyme, sage, fennel, salt, pepper, and cayenne over medium heat for about 5 minutes, or until the onion is soft.
- Add rinsed lentils and maple syrup. Cook 5 minutes to combine flavours. Gently press into a single layer.
- Top with a layer of shredded cheese.
- Whisk milk and eggs together. Pour over top slowly. Top with a layer of frozen kale puffs.
- Place uncovered casserole in the oven and bake for about 40 minutes, until the sides are bubbling, and the top is golden brown.
- Remove from oven and let it rest for 10 minutes.
- Garnish with chives and serve with hot sauce.

Black Bean & Vegan Sausage Grain-Free Burrito

Ingredients (6 servings):
- 1 tsp canola oil
- 1/2 white onion, diced
- 1/2 red bell pepper, diced
- 1 packet hot taco seasoning blend (or make your own seasoning)
- One 12-oz container Lightlife Plant-Based Ground
- Cooking spray
- 3 large eggs
- One 15 1/2-oz can black beans, drained and rinsed
- 6 Siete Cassava Flour Wraps
- 1/4 cup shredded cheddar cheese
- Hot sauce
- Fresh cilantro

Instructions:
- Take a medium skillet, heat the canola oil and sautée onion and bell pepper over medium-high heat. Stir occasionally, cooking for 3 minutes until onions are translucent and bell pepper is soft.
- Add taco seasoning and stir.

- Add Lightlife ground to pan and use a spoon to press into a single layer, chopping into small pieces. Cook for five to seven minutes, stirring occasionally until completely browned.
- In a separate small pan over medium heat, coat pan with cooking spray, add eggs, whisk into a scramble.
- Remove from heat.
- Heat cassava wraps a few seconds on the stovetop. To assemble the burrito, layer the Lightlife ground, scrambled eggs, black beans, and cheese.
- Top with hot sauce and fresh cilantro.
- Serve immediately or wrap and freeze for later.

Avocado Crispbreads with Everything Bagel Seasoning

Ingredients (2 servings):
- 4 Finn Crisp Thin Rye Crispbreads
- 1 small ripe avocado
- 2 tsp everything bagel seasoning
- 1 lemon wedge
- 2 radishes, thinly sliced
- Fresh dill, or other fresh herbs you have in fridge

Instructions:
- Cut avocado in half and remove pit.
- Slice it thinly and layer on top of each crispbread.
- Top each crispbread with the everything bagel seasoning, a squeeze of lemon juice, radish slices, and fresh dill.

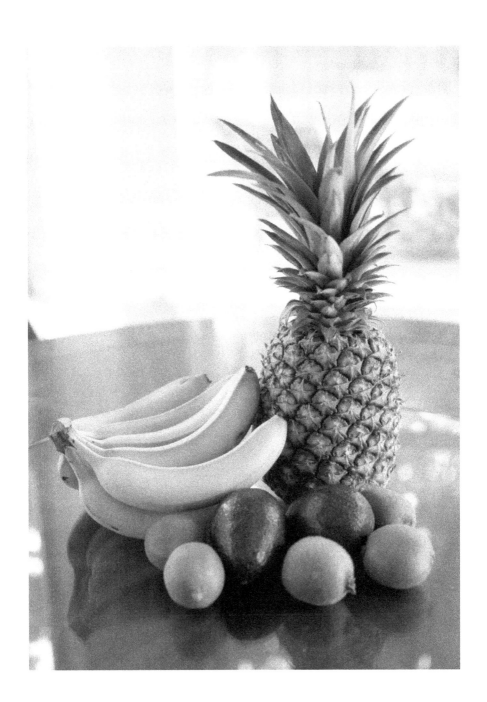

CHAPTER 5: LAUNCH RECIPES

Cilantro, corn and black bean salad

It is always a good idea to keep a couple of cans of corn and cans of black beans in the pantry. They are very versatile and quick options to add flavour and protein to a meal.

Ingredients (2 servings):
- Salad
- 1 cup of black beans
- ¼ cup of corn (low sodium and no sugar added)
- 2 cups of greens of your choice (ex: spring mix, spinach, or iceberg lettuce)
- ¼ green pepper or red peppers (sweet), diced
- ¼ red onion
- 2 tablespoons of chopped cilantro

Dressing:
- 1 tablespoon of olive oil
- Juice of one lime
- ¼ teaspoon of ground cumin
- ¼ teaspoon of sea salt
- Chopped cilantro (to taste)

Instructions:

- In a serving bowl, place the greens.
- Then, make the dressing. In a small bowl, mix all the ingredients together and set aside.
- In a large bowl, combine the black beans, corn, sweet peppers, and red onion. Once combined, add the dressing.
- Add the black beans mix to the serving bowl on top of the greens. Top with cilantro and serve.

Hummus Veggie Wrap

Wraps are easy and a way to make a quick lunch without spending too much time in the kitchen. If you are opting for vegan, vegan wraps exist! Sometimes, they hide in the frozen section, avoid your time and simply ask your store representative where you can find them in your local store.

Ingredients (1 servings):

- 1 Wraps (whole grains are usually a delicious option)
- ½ tomato, sliced
- ½ avocado, sliced
- 1/3 English cucumber, cut like sticks
- 1 tablespoons of hummus (you can try garlic hummus if you feel adventurous)

- Optional: 2 kalamata olives, pitted and halves

Instructions:
- Place the wrap on a plate and spread the hummus in the middle of the wrap.
- Add the tomatoes, cucumbers and avocado in the wrap (and olives if you picked that option).
- Close the wrap and enjoy now or store away for your lunch!

Vegetable and lentil soup

Soup is by far a family favourite during cold days of winter. This soup can be made in advance and stored for lunches.

Ingredients (4 servings):
- 2 Tbsp coconut oil (or water)
- 2 garlic cloves, minced
- 4 large carrots, sliced
- 2 stalks celery, sliced or diced
- 1 yellow onion, diced
- 4 cups of vegetable broth
- 1 small can of diced tomatoes (low sodium and no sugar added)
- 1/4 teaspoon sea salt

- 1/4 teaspoon black pepper
- 1 cup uncooked green or brown lentils (thoroughly rinsed and drained)

Instructions:
- In a large pot, over medium heat, add the oil or the water to the pot.
- When pot is hot, add the garlic, carrots, onions, and celery. Cook for 4 minutes.
- Add broth, tomatoes, and spices (salt and pepper) and slightly increase the heat. Once broth is simmering, add the lentils.
- Stir the lentils in broth and reduce the heat as soon as it starts simmering again.
- Let it cook, uncovered, for approximately 15 minutes (until the lentils are tender).
- You can serve now or store it in the fridge for up to 5 days. This recipe can also go in the freezer.

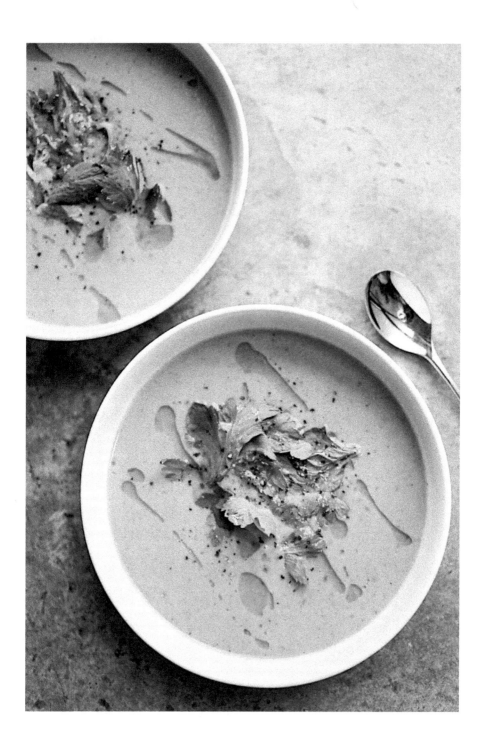

CHAPTER 6: DINNER RECIPES

Veggie and grain bowl

This recipe is versatile and allows you to mix and match with your favourite ingredients.

Ingredients (1 serving):
- 1 cup of cooked grains
- ½ cup of legumes
- 1 cup of veggies
- 2 tablespoons of nuts
- 2 tablespoons of dressing
- Optional: spices of your choice

Instructions:
- In a serving bowl, place grains, add the legumes and veggies, top with nuts, dressing and spices you like.

Rice and beans with plantains

This Costa Rican inspired dish is very filling and a great option that will please whole family! If it is your first-time trying plantains, make sure that the plantain is ripe. A ripe plantain is, unlike bananas, black and some yellow can be seen (but not green).

Ingredients (4 servings):

Rice:

- 1 cups of white rice
- 1 tablespoon of coconut oil (or oil of your choice)
- 1/2 yellow onion, chopped
- 1/4 cup celery, diced
- ½ sweet pepper, diced
- 1 carrot, diced
- 2 cloves of garlic, minced
- 2 cups of vegetable stock

Instructions:

- In a strainer, rinse the rice under cool water and set aside.
- Add the coconut oil to a medium-size pot and set at medium heat. Once the oil is ready, add the onions, celery, pepper, carrot and garlic. Cook for 2 minutes.
- Add rice to pot and stir. After stirring once, add the vegetable broth and bring to a boil.
- Once boiling, reduce the heat to low or simmer and cover the pot. Cook for about 15 minutes or until the rice is tender.

Beans:

- 1 tablespoon of coconut oil
- 1/2 cup diced onion
- 1 cloves of garlic, minced
- 1 tablespoon of tomato paste
- 1 bay leaf
- 2 cans of black beans, drain and rinse one can.
- 1 cup of vegetable broth
- 1 teaspoon of cumin
- 1/2 teaspoon of chili powder
- Juice of 1 lime
- Optional: cilantro, chopped

Instructions:

- Add the oil to a large skillet over medium heat. Once the oil is hot, add the onions and cook to translucent.
- Add garlic, tomato paste and bay leaf. Cook for thirty seconds.
- Add the black beans (the whole can and the drained beans) to the skillet. Mash some of the beans (about half of them).
- Add the broth, cumin and chili powder and cook for 10 minutes at low heat.

- When ready, turn off the heat and add the lime juice and cilantro (if using)
- Serve with Rice.

Plantain:

- 1 ripe plantain, peeled and sliced in 1" slices
- 1 tablespoons butter
- Honey

Instructions:

- Melt butter in a non-stick skillet over medium heat (be careful not to burn the butter).
- Add the plantains to the skillets so that they are in a single layer.
- Cook the plantain for around 3 minutes (you will see brown caramelized colour) and flip them to cook for 3 minutes on the other side.
- When a few seconds is left to cooking time, drizzle with honey and serve with your rice and bean dish.

Risotto with roasted veggies

Risotto is an Italian dish that takes time and patience. Make sure that you are ready to spend about an hour in the kitchen. It is extremely simple and is absolutely worth the wait because that dish is so delicious!

Ingredients (2 servings):

Roasted vegetables:

- 10 Brussels sprouts, cleaned and halves
- 2 Beets, peeled, cleaned and diced
- 4 garlic cloves, sliced
- 1 tablespoon of olive oil

Risotto:

- 4 cups chicken broth, divided
- 2 tablespoons coconut oil,
- ½ portobello mushrooms, diced
- 1 small yellow onion, diced
- 1 cup Arborio rice
- 1/3 cup dry white wine
- 1 tablespoons butter
- Ground pepper, to taste
- Salt, to taste

Instructions:

- Preheat the oven to 425 degrees.
- Meanwhile, in a large bowl, mix all the ingredients for the roasted vegetables.
- Transfer the vegetables to a prepared baking sheet.
- When over is ready, roast vegetables for 20 minutes.
- Warm vegetable broth in a sauce pan over low heat.
- Add coconut oil to a large sauce pan over medium heat.
- Add the mushrooms to the pan and let it cook for 2 minutes and then add the arborio rice.
- Stir the rice for about a minute and then add the dry wine. Stir until the wine is all absorbed.
- When there is no liquid in the skillet, add ½ cup of the vegetable broth, and stir often, until the broth is absorbed.
- Adding ½ cup of broth and wait until it's absorbed until you use all the broth in saucepan. This process should take about 20 minutes.
- When roasted vegetables are ready, pull out of oven.
- When rice is ready, divide in two and place in two plates. Add the roasted vegetables on top, salt and pepper to taste and enjoy as soon as it is ready or later in your lunch.

Snacks

Snacks for plant-based eaters can be as simple as a fruit or a vegetable. But sometimes we want a little more. Popcorn is also a great option for a good healthy snack. If you are a "snacker" be careful how much calories you consume, especially if it comes from sugar or sodium. Those extra calories can be a detriment to your health.

Almond stuffed date ingredients:
- 4 dry dates, pit removed
- 4 whole almonds

Instructions:
- Place an almond inside date (replacing pit) and eat!

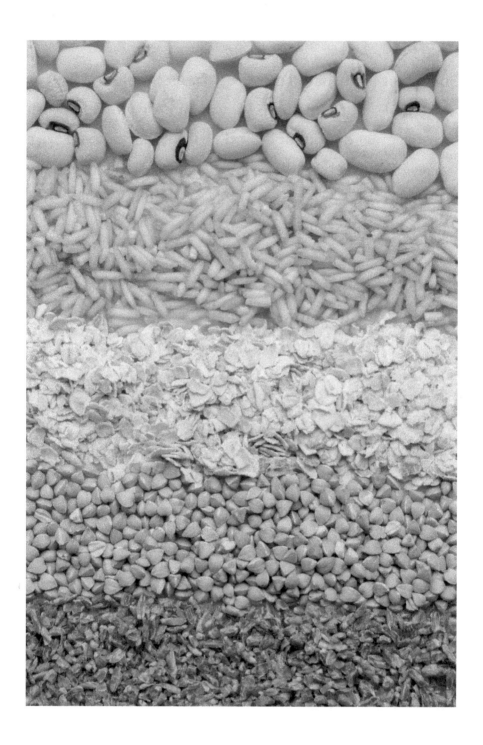

CHAPTER 7: ADDITIONAL TIPS FOR SUCCESS

Here are answers to questions that might be on your mind after reading the previous chapters.

What if I am invited to someone's place for dinner?
Well, if you are a flexitarian, that should not be an issue since you have allowed some flexibility in your nutrition plan for situations like this. If you are a vegetarian or pescatarian, there are usually an option on table, unless the person is making a meat lasagne, that would be difficult to opt out. In all cases, you might be able to prevent some uncomfortable situation and set you up for success by simply asking your host if you can bring a salad and if that tactic does not work, be honest. Compassion and honesty are the best policy! That could also be an opportunity for you to share why you have chosen this goal. Caution, don't be a preacher; no one likes to hear that what they are doing is wrong and what the other one is doing is better.

What if I am going out for a meal?

Be prepared! Always look at the restaurant menu before choosing where you eat. While plant-based meal options are more prominent than ever, it is not always on menu. If you forget to look at the menu in advance and end up in a place where you have no options, choose a garden salad, or ask for a menu item without the meat.

What if I eat meat by mistake?

As a plant-based eater, it might happen that you realize there is chicken in your wrap or beef in your salad. No big deal, you have eaten meat before. On the other hand, if you are going for the vegan option, you will need to do some research on what ingredients are vegan. Condiments like mayonnaise, Worcestershire or horseradish sauce may contain animal product. Make sure that you are well informed on products that are vegan-friendly.

Is potato chips plant-based eating?

Yes, potato chips are technically a plant-based food but beware of junk food! It is a highly processed food that often contains a large amount of sodium.

If you stick to the recommendations of the daily intake of 2300 mg of sodium and 50 mg of sugar, you will quickly realize that eating junk food is unsustainable since a bag of chips (party size) contains about 2550 mg of sodium and 15 g of sugar. A 4 oz chocolate bar can contain 80 mg of sodium, 56 g of sugar. Add a can of regular soda (or pop) to mix and you now have an additional 30 mg of sodium and 41 g of sugar.

What about milk?

Studies show that humans stop producing the enzyme that metabolizes the lactose in breast milk after an early age in life. That said, it is fair to say we become lactose intolerant very early in our childhood. It is estimated that 75% of us are lactose intolerant. Yet, many people in our country, consume cow milk. Choosing a plant-based nutrition can be an opportunity for you to plant-based milk like almond milk, coconut milk, rice milk, etc. Many options are now available at most grocery stores.

What about fat?

Fat is a little bit harder to explain and a bit more complex to understand. As you have heard, there is good fat and bad fat.

The number one rule with fat is to stay away from trans-fat, as soon as you see it on a label in the grocery store, put that item back on the shelf. A general rule is that no more than 20–30% of calories should come from fat. The good news is that eating more vegetables and fruits can reduce the amount of fat intake.

What about physical fitness? And mental health?
As mentioned earlier, physical fitness plays an important part in health and weight loss. With plant-based nutrition, you will likely find yourself having more energy and will be motivated to be more active. Do not fall into the trap of committing to something you do not enjoy. According to a study, 63% of gym members do not use their membership. Find something you enjoy doing and do more of it. Also, do not stop yourself from being active because you do not have a full hour a day to dedicate to it. A quick 20 minutes of high-intensity interval training is enough to make you sweat. If you are already active, pay attention to changes of your body during gym sessions and after, you might want to increase your plant-based protein intake.

And mental health?

According to research plant-based eaters showed fewer signs of depression and mental illness than omnivores. There is much more research to be done and certainly some aspects to consider (like sugar intake) but researches are very promising. The best way to know is to try it and see how you feel.

CHAPTER 8: THE INDISPENSABLE BENEFITS OF A PLANT-BASED DIET

Vegetables are a source of nutrients and fibers essential for a healthy diet. It is important to take them daily because they help in the treatment and prevention of diseases. We often wonder if vegetables and vegetables are synonymous. Vegetable means the vegetable product grown in garden and then harvested. The word "vegetable" - on the other hand - is a gastronomical nutritional term which indicates a "category of vegetable" according to the parts of plant (leaves, roots, etc.) used in nutrition.

Vegetables, in fact, are not a homogeneous group of foods because their structure depends on the different parts of the plants.

- Some of the vegetables are roots (beet, carrot, celery, radish, turnip) used for soups and salads. The only exception is horseradish which has a kind of bitter taste and is more used as a condiment.
- Bulbs (yellow or red onion, leek, garlic, shallots, and chives) can be used for their taste in various dishes, usually cut, chopped or sliced. Onions, shallots and leeks can be used raw in salads.

- Leafy vegetables (like lettuce, radicchio, watercress, spinach, arugula) are used in salads and as garnish of dishes and in some cases, for example in spinach, cooked.
- Among flowers or inflorescences of vegetables like broccoli, cauliflower, Brussels sprouts, cabbage, red cabbage, are typical vegetables, used raw, cooked, marinated or as ingredients for different dishes, also used in salads; other varieties are boiled or steamed.
- Fruiting vegetables (avocados, cucumbers, peppers, tomatoes, eggplant, pumpkins zucchini) are fruits in various stages of ripeness containing seeds inside. Some seeds are edible, while seeds of others must be removed to be ready for use. They can be used raw and in salads, they are base of many sauces, soups and stews.
- Stems and sprouts (like green or white asparagus, artichokes, celery, fennel, bean sprouts) have a wide range of uses. Celery and sprouts, for example, can be used raw in salads, while it is common to cook asparagus and artichokes.
- Pods and seeds (like broad beans, corn, peas, sweet peas/mangetout, rice) to be consumed are always cooked.

- Tubers (sweet potato, potato, jerusalem artichokes) also always cooked.

Vegetables, despite being so different have (except seeds and tubers), common nutritional characteristics.

The importance of a daily, constant intake of vegetables in our nutrition is represented by a series of nutritional principles they provide us with, for example, a good source of dietary fiber. This has no nutritional or energetic value, but it is also important for regulation of physiological body functions.

Fiber is made up, of complex carbohydrates, for the most part, not directly usable by human body. They are divided in two big groups: some of these compounds (cellulose, hemicellulose and lignin) are insoluble in water and act on the functioning of the gastrointestinal tract, delaying the gastric emptying, facilitating the transit in the intestine of the alimentary bolus and the evacuation of stools. Other compounds (pectins, gums, mucilages) are soluble in the water - in which they form resistant gels which coat walls of bowel - and regulate the absorption of some nutrients (for example sugars and fats) reducing and slowing them down.

Thus, contributing to the control of the level of glucose and cholesterol in blood. Vegetables provide essential vitamins and mineral salts: for example, tomatoes provide vitamin C, carrots, green leafy vegetables pro-vitamin A.

It is also important to remember folates, vitamins in which leafy vegetables are rich and which - together with B vitamins - can contribute to reduce level of homocysteine in blood, a known risk factor for cardiovascular diseases. They are also an important source of mineral salts (green leafy vegetables are rich in calcium and iron, potato, and tomato in potassium) even though absorption of the latter is usually lower than that of the same minerals contained in foods of animal origin. The consumption of vegetables can also ensure a significant intake of selenium and zinc which are part of the antioxidant defence systems of body.

Other important substances provided by vegetables and fruits, although present in relatively small quantities, are components that can play an important protective action mainly of antioxidant type by contrasting the action of free radicals, which can alter the structure of cell membranes and of the genetic material (DNA). Among these we find:

- Carotenoids (the yellow, orange and red pigments in which vegetables are rich - for the presence of beta-carotene - and red ones such as tomatoes – thanks to the presence of lycopene).
- Phenolic compounds.
- Tocopherols (especially in green leafy vegetables).

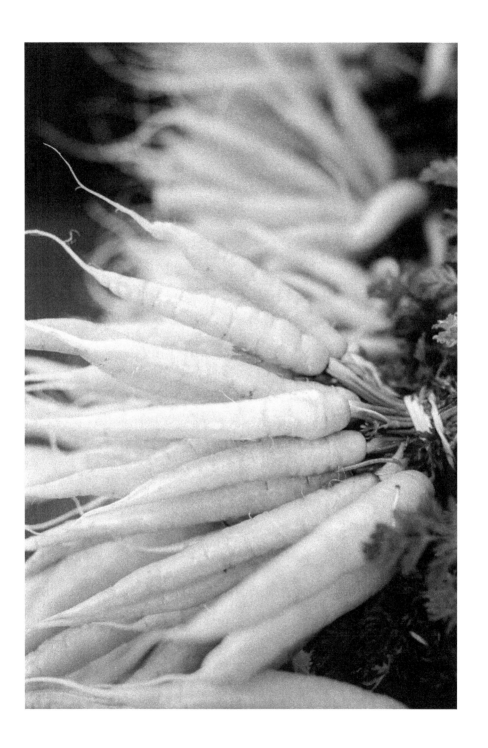

CHAPTER 9: THE SECRET TRICKS TO BRING MORE PROTEIN

About vegetarian and plant-based diets it has been said everything and the opposite of everything: in addition to the classic false myths to be debunked, the main subject of discussions concerns, both for the bad and for the good, the contribution, or not, of nutrients and effects, healthy or not, on the organism and health in general. Whatever your opinion is, one thing is for sure: just like any other diet cannot be taken lightly and it requires attention and preparation.

My advice is therefore to deepen argument and to contact a nutritionist doctor if you decide to undertake this diet. As we have seen, if you decide to become vegan or vegetarian, especially in the preparatory phase and in the transition from an omnivorous diet to a meatless diet, it may be useful to take some precautions to maintain a balance and not to run into deficiencies. One of the main problems of those who start a vegan or vegetarian diet is how to replace meat proteins.

While always stressing the importance of medical support, a bit of foresight and a commitment to maintaining a varied and balanced diet, I would like to recommend ten vegetable sources of protein, which can therefore be a good starting point and can give you greater peace of mind when facing this important change:

1. LEGUMES: ABOVE ALL SOY, LUPINS AND LENTILS

Nutritional tables say it: legumes are the richest vegetable source of protein in nature, surpassing even meat. To those who tell you that they need a good steak for protein intake, you can therefore reply that a good plate of cereals and lentils wins over everything.

2. CEREALS: ABOVE ALL SPELT AND QUINOA
The most recommended cereals are whole grains. It is also important the so called "protein complementation", that is matching of cereals and legumes to increase assimilation of amino acids.

3. DRIED FRUIT

Dried fruit, in addition to being practical and convenient to carry and eat as a snack, can be chopped, and added to salads, sauces and other culinary preparations, just think of the many variants of Italian pesto, often made with pine nuts, walnuts and almonds. Just think that 100 grams of shelled almonds can contain up to 20 grams of protein. Of course, it is important to pay attention to the quantities: these are still caloric foods, even though they contain protein, and only small quantities are needed for the right nutritional intake.

4. SPIRULIN ALGA

There is no vegetarian who does not know the spirulina seaweed, which can be bought dried in leaves or powder form, especially in organic food stores, or taken as a supplement. Spirulina is in fact an alga particularly rich in vegetable proteins, rich in amino acids easily assimilated by the body.

In kitchen it can be used mostly as an addition to first or second courses, broths, or soups (if you need tips, in the past we have explained how to cook seaweed!)

5. SOY DERIVATIVES: TOFU AND TEMPEH

The most famous and easily available tofu and less known alternative tempeh are products derived from soy, both very rich in vegetable proteins with 8/10 grams per 100 grams. Mistakenly called "vegetable cheeses", even though they are not dairy products, they can represent an excellent alternative to meat, and therefore provide you with many creative ideas for your second courses.

6. SPROUTS

Most sprouts contain 20-35% protein, but they are also an excellent source of enzymes and vitamins and in general are a concentrate of active nutrients. Sprouts can be an excellent ingredient for salads or first courses, very used for oriental dishes, to be consumed both raw and cooked. Particularly recommended are lentil and azuki sprouts.

7. SEEDS, ABOVE ALL HEMP, CHIA AND PUMPKIN, SUNFLOWERS

Seeds, in cooking, can be eaten as snacks, or inside sweet and salty snacks, but also added, even finely chopped, to salads and various culinary preparations such as bread, cookies, first and second courses.

8. DEHYDRATED APRICOTS

A good source of vegetable proteins is also constituted by fruit and by dehydrated apricots. Apricots can be a snack, preferably consumed together with dried fruits such as almonds. They can be used in recipes for sweets as well as in sauces to accompany main courses and cheeses.

9. VEGETABLES

Those with a higher intake of vegetable proteins are raw spinach and boiled cabbage, but also artichokes, peppers, asparagus and potatoes.

10. VEGETABLE MILK

There are many varieties of vegetable milk, with higher and lower protein content. Vegetable milk in cooking does the same as cow milk, in fact it can be consumed as a beverage or used for sauces, béchamel, mayonnaise and any other preparation, even "cheese". However, pay attention to the possible addition of sugar and in general keep in mind these beverages can be naturally more or less bitter and therefore to be used for different recipes.

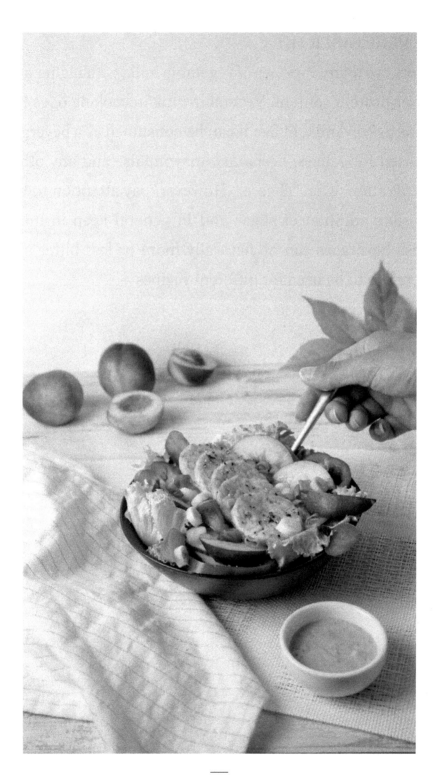

CHAPTER 10: 5 REASONS WHY BEING VEGETARIAN IS GOOD FOR THE PLANET

When we talk about plant-based eating, often first mental association I hear people make is about the healthy aspect of this choice, as well as the animal rights aspect. But it is not only love for animals and for a healthy diet that pushes vegetarians to take this step: a topic still largely neglected by the media, and consequently by common opinion, is the environmental impact of the animal food industry.

Let's summarize everything in five good reasons why being vegetarian is good for the planet.

#1 - WE CAN STEM GROWTH OF MEAT PRODUCTION AND ENVIRONMENTAL IMPACT

According to statistics, meat production levels are set to rise from 309 million tons in 2013 to 465 million in 2050, when the world's population will have surpassed 9 billion. We have already witnessed in last 50 years an impressive increase in consumption, which has grown 5 times more than before, which has been matched by an increase in the number of animals raised.

A deterioration in the quality of meat and in general the industrialization of the livestock sector. Our food choices have a dramatic impact on planet: according to a research carried out by the UN*, meat farming is responsible for 18% of gas and 37% of methane emissions: just think that omnivores contribute to greenhouse gas emissions 7 times more than vegans. Furthermore, raising animals for food is one of the three activities that contribute most to the world's most serious environmental problems. It is worth pausing to reflect on how much animal products and intensive farming, dramatically affect global atmospheric emissions and natural balances and biodiversity.

#2 - WE CAN ENCOURAGE THE SPREAD OF MORE SUSTAINABLE LIVESTOCK FARMING

One might think vegetarians sensitive to environmental issues have a utopian hope to live, one day, in a world of vegetarians. This is not the case at all: what is hoped for, in most cases, is above an awareness of the characteristics and environmental impact of intensive livestock farming and a reduction, if not even the disappearance, of farming.

The "average vegetarian" knows well difference between intensive farming and family or sustainable farming, i.e., organic, or free-range. Intensive farming uses industrial and scientific techniques to obtain the maximum amount of product at the minimum cost and using the minimum amount of space, typically with use of special machinery and veterinary drugs. Focusing on environmental aspect, it should be remembered that intensive farming not only requires a large and dramatic use of natural resources but also a use of chemicals of poor quality and therefore highly polluting.

#3 - WE CAN SAVE THE FORESTS

Thanks to an estimate by Greenpeace we discover that due to animal farming an average of one hectare of Amazonian forest is lost every 8 seconds. Production of meat, of palm oil, sugar, paper has significantly increased deforestation. Over the last 10 years, efforts are being made to make consumers understand that meat consumption is one of the main culprits in felling of 70% of forests, particularly in the Amazon, the largest rainforest in the world.

#4 - WE CAN CURB THE CONSUMPTION OF WATER RESOURCES

Animal farming requires an inordinate and impressive use of water resources. First of all, water is needed to water the animals: think that a dairy cow drinks over 200 liters of water per day, a pig twenty and a sheep ten. Water is also needed for the cleaning and maintenance of farms as well as for the cultivation of fodder and for slaughter process.

#5 - LESS INTENSIVE FARMING = LESS SUFFERING FOR ANIMALS

I have left the animal rights aspect for last, but I would like to point out that it is often from the knowledge of intensive farming that a greater environmentalist attention can arise and, as an ultimate consequence, a greater attention in the selection and consumption of meat. There are all over the world many animal associations that for years have been fighting to shed light on the critical conditions of animals and their suffering: among cases of mistreatment reported have emerged practices such as amputations, lack of air and light, muscle atrophy caused by lack of space and other atrocious practices far worse.

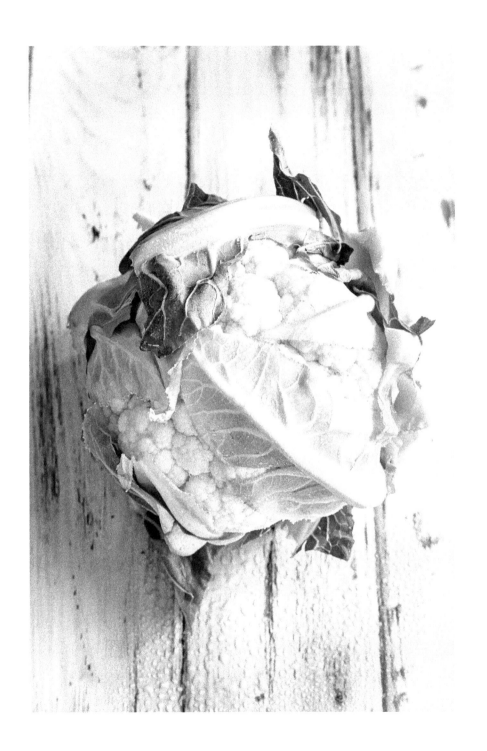

CHAPTER 11: THE 5 PRINCIPAL REASONS TO START PLANT-BASED NUTRITION

The plant-based diet has been shown to be beneficial to the heart. Research conducted a few years ago by a team at the University of Oxford found that individuals who do not eat meat or fish have a 32% lower risk of heart disease. This would be attributed to the fact that vegetarians, in general, have lower body mass indexes (BMI) and fewer cases of diabetes, in addition to far lower cholesterol levels and a more regular blood pressure.

Plant-based diet promotes weight loss, even without heavy training, exaggerating with exercise and without counting calories, according to a meta-analysis published in Journal of the Academy of Nutrition and Dietetics. According to the results found by researchers at Physicians Committee for Responsible Medicine, individuals who went on a diet following a plant-based diet lost about 10 pounds. Not just any plant-based diet, however, recommended diet should be based mainly on whole grains, legumes, vegetables and fruits, even better if organically grown.

It seems then that the vegetarian diet is good for the mood. This was revealed by a research published in the journal Psychosomatic Medicine, which once again turns spotlight on carotenoids, antioxidants capable of eliminating free radicals, helping immune system. Experts noted that those who consumed three or more servings a day of fruits and vegetables were more optimistic than those who did not get to two, this is because they found higher amounts of beta-carotene in the blood.

Being rich in vitamins, minerals and fiber, the vegetarian diet helps to feel fitter and keep the body young. This type of diet also allows us to introduce less hormones and the antibiotics into our bodies, which are increasingly present especially in the meat derived from intensive farming and farmed fish. To recap the benefits that the vegetarian diet offers are:

- Helps heart health
- Promotes weight loss (if well balanced)
- Improves mood
- Promotes longevity
- Minimizes intake of hormones and antibiotics

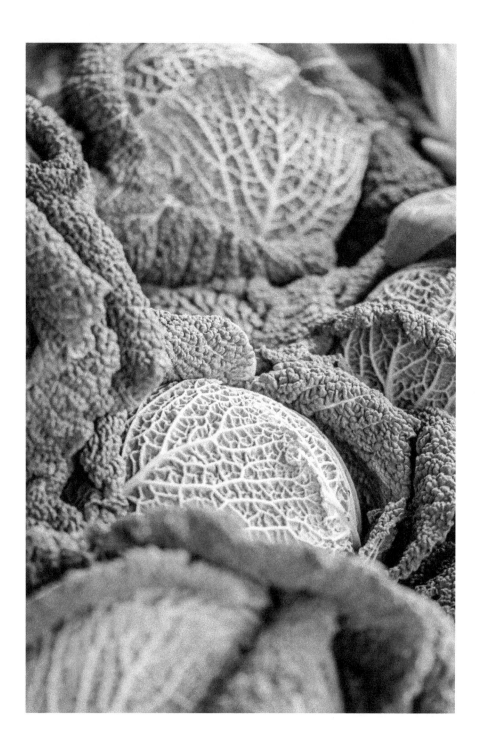

CHAPTER 12: HOW TO STICK TO PLANT-BASED EATING

Plant-based eating can be for everyone, the main idea is not to diet or remove something from your nutrition but more about adding more vegetables, fruits, nuts, whole grains, and legumes. For those of you who love their steak or beef burgers occasionally, you do not have to completely eliminate animal-based food, but you can certainly reduce it by making more meals that are plant-based.

You can stick to a plant-based nutrition by following these two simple steps:

#Step 1: Have a grocery list
T stick to plant-based eating, have a grocery list. Here's one we made for you:

Fruits/Vegetables
- Apples
- Avocado
- Bananas
- Berries
- Blueberries

- Grapefruit
- Grapes
- Lemons/Limes
- Oranges
- Pears
- Tomatoes
- Asparagus
- Beets
- Broccoli
- Brussels sprouts
- Carrots
- Cauliflower
- Celery
- Corn
- Cucumbers
- Garlic
- Lettuce/Greens
- Mushrooms
- Onions
- Squash Sweet Peppers
- Jalapenos
- Chilis
- Potatoes
- Spinach

- Squash
- Zucchini
- Sweet potatoes

Grains/Legumes/Herbs and spices/Other
- Rice
- Farro
- Quinoa
- Tabbouleh
- Couscous
- Barley
- Rolled Oat
- Chickpeas
- Pinto Beans
- Lentils
- Split Peas
- Mung beans
- Red kidney beans
- Soybeans
- Black beans
- Basil
- Pepper
- Cilantro
- Cinnamon
- Cumin

- Curry
- Garlic
- Ginger
- Mint
- Oregano
- Parsley
- Pepper
- Salt
- Vegan sour cream
- Vegan mayonnaise
- Vegan bread & wraps
- Whole grain mustard
- Bran cereals
- Honey or Maple syrup
- Peanut butter
- Almond milk
- Coconut milk
- Coconut oil
- Olive oil
- Hummus
- Tahini

#Step 2: Plan Your Meals in Advance

Here are our favourite ideas for breakfast, lunch, dinner:

Breakfast

- Bran cereals with bananas and plant-base milk (this will be a winner for your fiber intake).
- Oatmeal in a jar.
- Vegan bread with natural peanut butter and no sugar added jam.
- Fruit salad.
- Lunch.
- Salads.
- Wraps.
- Soups.
- Dinner.
- Veggie Burger with sweet potato fries.
- Vegetable, black beans and rice stir fries.
- Grain bowls.
- Grains with roasted vegetables.

The more you will be prepared, the easier it will be to stick to a plant-based nutrition.

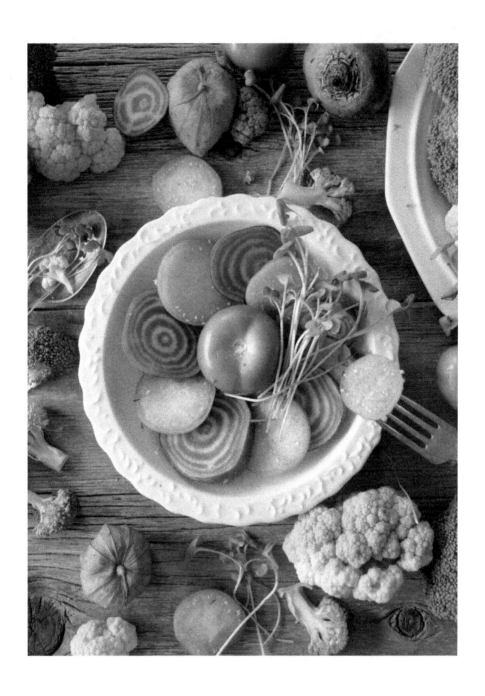

CHAPTER 13: HOW TO LOSE WEIGHT ON PLANT-BASED NUTRITION

In general, individuals who are on a plant-based nutrition tend to consume fewer calories than people who consume animal protein since most of their calories are coming from healthier options and fewer calories per weight. Not all plant-based food is healthy, here is a few suggestions to increase change of losing weight on plant-based lifestyle nutrition.

❖ *Eat More Fruits and Vegetables*

Doctors and experts in nutrition all across the world agree that an insufficient consumption of fruits and vegetables contribute to obesity epidemic and chronic disease related to poor nutrition. Plant-based eating means that you have a large proportion of your meal that comes from plant-based food. To fight weight gain, reach the recommended daily intake of 400 g of fruits and vegetable.

❖ *Reduce Your Sodium*

Sodium might be considered a plant-based food but there is a strong warning to decrease our consumption so that we do not exceed the requirements of 2300 mg of sodium consumption daily. So, it is important to understand that plant-based food does not always mean healthy food. According to some research, individuals who eat a plant-based nutrition with reduce sodium consumption (2300 mg per day) showed a reduction in the blood pressure and increased weight loss.

❖ *Reduce Your Sugar*

Sugar is other plant-based food to beware of. It is highly recommended to stick to less than 50 g of sugar a day. We challenge you to start looking at the labels of the food you eat daily and identify amount of sugar intake you get from those foods. Many companies hide the ingredient by using multiple names to describe sugar added, they use at least sixty names for sugar on labels. By reducing your sugar intake, you can increase your chance of losing weights and staying healthy while preventing chronic disease.

Reading labels can be difficult, look for the word sugar on the nutrition label, you will be able to identify how many grams of sugar is in the product.

While thousands of researches demonstrate health benefit of consuming vegetables as a way to be healthy, many still refuse to change their nutrition to increase our quality of life. Too many people believe that exercising, medication and supplements are sufficient to maintain health. Meanwhile, experts in the field of health and wellness say that weight management is about 75% nutrition and 25% exercise.

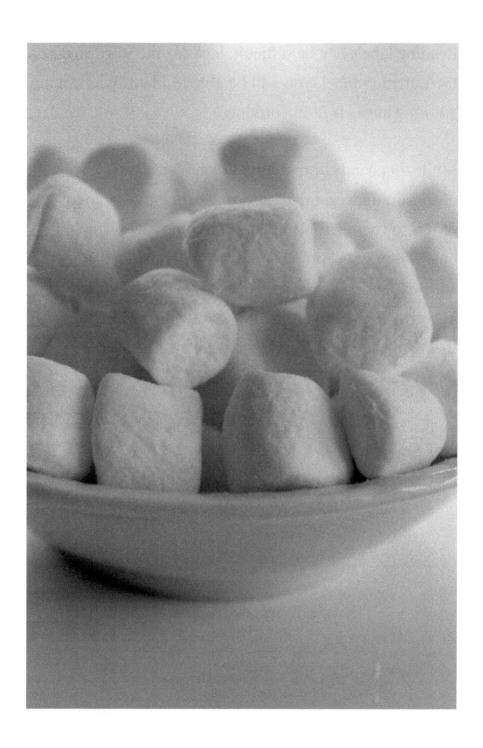

CHAPTER 14: ECO-SUSTAINABILITY AND FOOD AWARENESS OF PLANT-BASED DIET

If you are used to do your shopping by putting in your cart only special offers and refined foods loaded with fats and sugars, it will be difficult to take this step... But it is not impossible. It is necessary to learn to always read labels of products, both as ingredients and as origin and processing of the same. Only by really knowing what you put on our table - such as origin or nutritional values - you can really understand if it is suitable for this diet. And that is not all: consuming fresh foods means following seasonality.

In October we eat pumpkin, in July watermelon, it cannot be otherwise: pretending to eat strawberries in December and chestnuts in June creates need to force nature's hand, with intensive cultivations in greenhouses and processing to preserve food beyond the right season.

This focus on following nature's rhythm, to avoid forcing by industries, is good for the environment, although plant-based is more about health than the purely ethical choice of veganism.

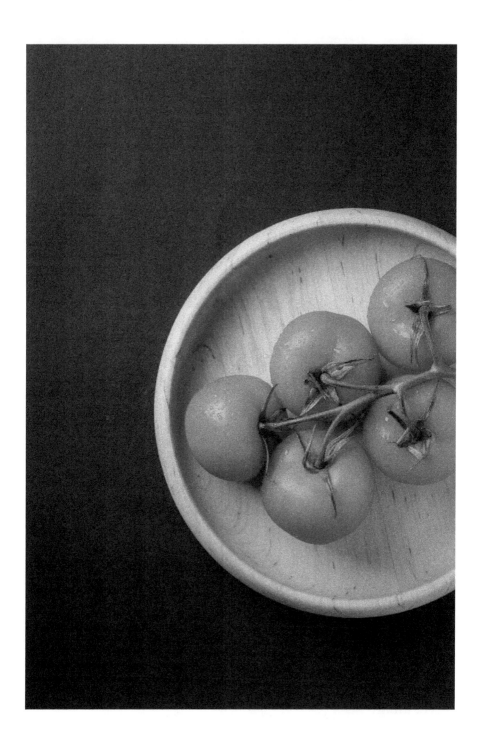

CHAPTER 15: THE 3 STEPS TO EASLY START EAT HEALTHY

Those who are thinking of switching to a vegetarian diet to improve their health will be happy to discover another nice and pleasant effect of plant-based eating: it is delicious and fun to discover and experiment with these new foods.

A plant-based meal can be as familiar as a plate of pasta with tomato and basil, as relaxing as a legume soup, or as nice as a plate of beans and red radicchio typical of the Mediterranean cuisine. Transitioning to a vegetarian diet is far easier than people think. Many people, vegetarian or carnivore, usually use a limited number of recipes.

An average family usually uses at most 12 dishes cyclically. So, you can use this simple, 3-steps method to switch to enjoyable, easy-to-prepare vegetarian menus.

#Step 1 - Add:

Identify some already vegetarian dishes that you enjoy and begin to consume them more frequently. Many soups from our Mediterranean tradition are already vegetarian or can be easily adapted with some adjustments (e.g., avoiding lard in pasta and beans and using vegetable stock cubes in soups). Other common dishes include steamed vegetables, minestrone, pasta or rice with vegetables or legumes.

#Step 2 - Substitute:

Focus on a few recipes you already know how to cook and make a vegetarian version: for example, a pasta carbonara can easily be transformed by replacing the egg with white tofu and the bacon with cubes of seitan and colouring it yellow with a little curry or saffron. Meat stew or sauce can be transformed by replacing the meat with seitan stew or meatballs or soy granola. Introduce these kinds of dishes more frequently into your diet as well.

#Third and final step – Learn:

Buy yourself a good recipe book and try to experiment with the recipes that most appeal to you, until you identify at least 3-5 recipes that most appeal to you in terms of taste and simplicity of preparation.

In this way - and with minimal effort - you can obtain an assortment of vegetarian dishes sufficient to satisfy palate without risking boredom. At this point it will also be easy to adapt your breakfast: favour whole grains, to be eaten with fresh fruit, hazelnut cream or with vegetables and tofu cubes if you know you will be skipping lunch. Replace milk from cow with soy or rice milk.

The next step, but essential, towards healthy eating is to strive to "simplify" as much as possible foods you consume, preferring foods in their original and natural state, "as gathered" (cereals, whole grain bread and pasta, legumes, steamed vegetables) to "processed" foods (like meatballs, seitan, hamburgers, sausages, sauces, condiments, canned vegetables, etc.). That should be reserved for "emergency" situations.

If you know how to organize yourself it is quite easy to prepare in a short time a certain quantity of legumes, cereals and vegetables which can then be used as a base for various dishes for several days.

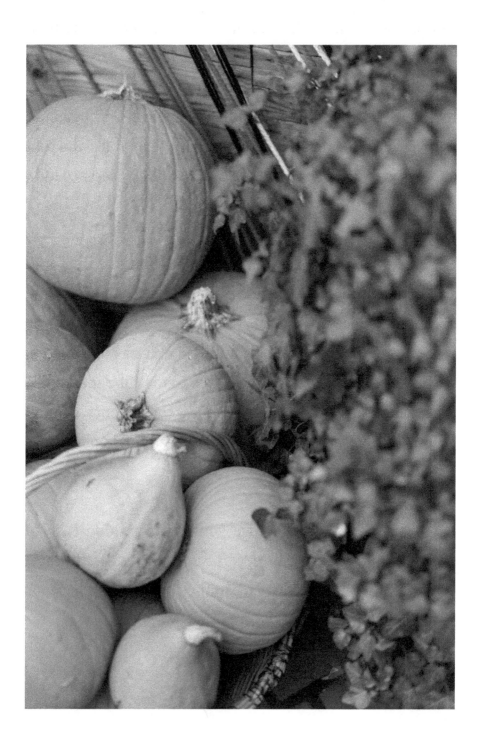

CONCLUSION

Plant-based eating can be for everyone, the main idea is not to "diet" or remove something from your nutrition but more about adding more vegetables, fruits, nuts, whole grains, and legumes. For those of you who love their steak or burgers once in a while, you don't have to completely eliminate animal-based food but you can certainly reduce it by making more meals that are plant-based.

As you have seen from the research, there is a strong advantage not to surpass daily intake recommendations for sugar, sodium and protein. This is the optimal way to avoid health issues and prevent chronic diseases. While exercising is important, nutrition is probably the number one reason why we have so much obesity in our nation. Not knowing what to eat and difficulty reading labels has led us to be confused about what to eat or not to eat. The best approach is a balanced nutrition with a lot of variety and refrain from overindulging.

Now it is time to put your learning into action. First, pick a day when you will start you plant-based eating, then select your meals (breakfast, lunch, dinner recipes), go shopping and get your grocery items and implement the change!

If it seems like a big change for you, try once a week for the first month and gradually move to twice a week, three times a week, etc. Remember, slow and steady is a great approach to change habits but mostly to make them stick. Plant-based eating is not a diet but a way of living so have fun with it!

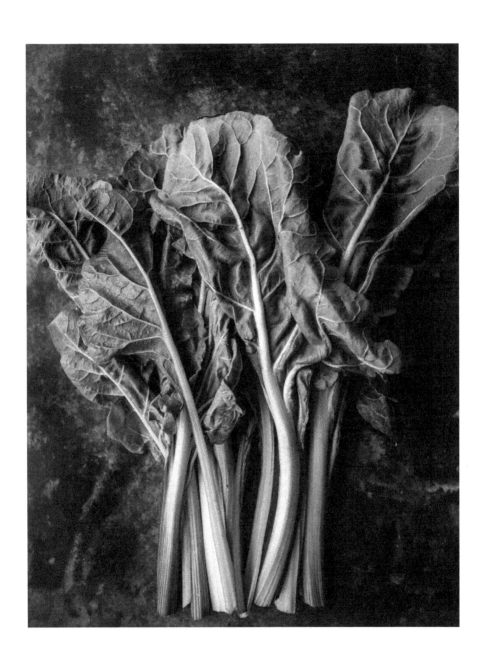